SWISS MICRONIZED Flower Pollen

"The Most Concentrated, Nutrient-Rich Food in the World"

A report from The National Life Extension Research Institute

Other books by the author on related health topics:

Coenzyme Q10: A Key to Unleashing Powerful Cellular Energy

Discovered: Nature's Secret Fountains of Youth

The Olive Leaf: Unequalled Immune Support for Health and Longevity

Swiss Micronized Flower Pollen "The Most Concentrated, Nutrient-Rich Food in the World"

Seventh Printing

Copyright ©1999 by
National Life Extension Research Institute
1675 East Main St. #P303
Kent, Ohio 44240

Additional copies of this book may be obtained for $5.00 postpaid.

All rights reserved. No part of this publication may be reproduced, stored in a retrieval system, or transmitted, in any form by any means, electronic, mechanical, photocopying, recording, digital or otherwise, without the prior written permission of the publisher. Printed in the United States of America.

IMPORTANT:

The information herein is intended to help you make informed decisions about your diet and health, not to substitute for any treatment that may have been prescribed by your physician. If you suspect that you have a medical problem, we urge you to seek competent medical help. Keep in mind that nutritional needs vary from person to person, depending on age, sex, health status and total diet. Because there may be some individual risks involved, the publisher and researchers are not responsible for any adverse effects or consequences resulting from the use or misuse of any of the suggestions, preparations or procedures in this Report.

These statements have not been evaluated by the Food and Drug Administration. The information is not intended to diagnose, treat, cure or prevent any disease but rather is intended solely for nutritional use. A testimonial reflects the personal experience of one person. Individual results can and do vary.

Table of Contents

7	**INTRODUCTION**
9	**CHAPTER 1** Pollen as the Perfect Food
15	**CHAPTER 2** Two Types of Pollen
25	**CHAPTER 3** Pollen and the Prostate
35	**CHAPTER 4** Pollen and Allergies
41	**CHAPTER 5** Pollen and Athletics
47	**CHAPTER 6** Pollen and Good Health
57	**CHAPTER 7** Scientific Information on Pollen
65	**CHAPTER 8** The History of Flower Pollen

71	**CHAPTER 9**
	Clinical Studies and Anecdotal Reports
83	**APPENDIX A**
	Chemical Analysis of Flower Pollen
89	**APPENDIX B**
	Nutritional Analysis of Pollen
93	**REFERENCES**
95	**BIBLIOGRAPHY**

INTRODUCTION

Milestones in the field of medicine are usually larger-than-life and quite noteworthy. One might recall in this regard the discovery of penicillin, or the first heart transplant surgery by Dr. Christian Barnard.

Important discoveries in nutrition herald much the same attention. Gyorgi's discovery of Vitamin C, and the relatively recent classification of Coenzyme Q10 come to mind as significant events.

Ranking at the top with all of these is the nutritional powerhouse, Swiss Micronized Flower Pollen.

Unknown prior to 1970, this single supplement has taken Europe and Asia by storm. From its humble beginnings, it now fills the shelves of hundreds of pharmacies worldwide.

Sadly, most Americans have not yet had the opportunity to benefit from this potent life-giving substance.

On a personal note, flower pollen helped me win my weary and tiresome battle against a long-standing prostate problem, and lifelong hayfever allergies. For me, it is now one of those "never run out, must-have" supplements.

Join me now on a delightful journey as we share together what certainly must be considered nature's most perfect food — Swiss Micronized Flower Pollen.

Robert Concoby
Director of Research

Chapter 1

Pollen as the "Perfect Food"

The father of Medicine, Hippocrates, reportedly once stated, "Let your food be your medicine and your medicine be your food." Almost since the beginning of time, man has used pollen as a high-quality food. One of man's earliest foods was pollen. Cave drawings show honey hunters harvesting this food. The Bible, Roman writings, and other early narratives refer to the benefits of honey and pollen. Maimonides, a Hebrew physician to the Sultan of Egypt in the 13th century made reference to pollen as being a good tonic. In the early 13th century, Ibn el-Beithar described pollen as beneficial for the stomach, bowels and heart.[1] Homer referred to it as "the food of kings," and guests in Roman homes were welcomed with the words, "Here is honey and pollen, provided by the gods, to protect your health."[2]

In the Orient, honey and pollen were used as a supplement to the diet. It is even believed that John the Baptist of the Bible ate pollen with honey as a mainstay of his diet. To early civilizations in China, Greece, Egypt and elsewhere, honey and pollen were natural sources of food and nutrition.

Today, many people the world over recognize the value of pollen for good health, good eating, and its healthy qualities. It well deserves its reputation as nature's most perfect food.

Pollen is high in protein, low in fat, and contains an incredible wealth of vitamins, minerals and other nutrients.

> **Pollen helps the body adapt to stress and fight fatigue as well as stimulate its natural immune system.**

Pollen is unique in that it contains many biofactors to help maintain and improve health. Pollen helps the body adapt to stress and fight fatigue as well as stimulate its natural immune system.

Research into the anti-pathogenic characteristics of pollen yielded exciting results. Various viruses, bacteria, yeasts and fungi are neutralized by pollen or derivative products.[3]

Researchers have found that a diet including pollen has high antioxidant power rivaling vitamin E. Sociologists and scientists studying populations with advanced, old-age members have found that a longer life of vigor and health can many times be traced largely to a diet high in fiber and pollen.

Researchers in Switzerland, Sweden, Germany, England and Belgium have found that pollen contains certain nutritional factors important to help relieve prostate problems such as benign prostatic hyperplasia and hypertrophy, urinary dysfunction and abnormal growth in hormone-insensitive cells.

Professor Alin Caillas, French agriculturist and Laureate of the Academy of Agriculture, reports that 35 grams of pollen daily can fulfill most of the nutritional requirements for an average person. About half that amount, 20 grams, provides the complete minimum protein (amino acids) that a human body needs. Half of pollen's protein is in the form of free amino acids, which can be assimilated immediately by the body.[2]

Pollen ranks higher overall in nutrients than any other food. Pollen has more protein than beef (as high as 35% protein) with much greater digestibility, and outranks the two most nutritious vegetables —tomatoes and cabbage.[1]

Chapter 2

Two Types of Pollen

UNPROCESSED BEE POLLEN - THE LESSER POLLEN

Many centenarians in the world worked as beekeepers. In so doing, they keep the dark honey for themselves — it's a far richer source of bee pollen. They know that queen bees grow three times larger and live many times longer with incredible fertility compared to the genetically identical worker bees. This occurs because they are fed a pollen food called "royal jelly" from the time they are born. The worker bees make royal jelly by taking pollen and mixing it with special enzymes, with the resulting liquid being royal jelly.

Notwithstanding the opinions of these beekeepers, bee pollen is actually a lesser-quality food. There are a number of reasons for this which merit further discussion.

It is impossible to precisely control what bees harvest — they may gather pollen from a plant that may cause an allergic reaction. To ingest bee pollen that contains allergens will perhaps cause an adverse response in an allergic individual.

The quality of ordinary bee pollen can be downgraded by the level of contamination from bee wings, legs, fly eggs, rodent hair, dung and other foreign matter. Harmful physiological responses may occur from these pollutants.

Of even more importance, however, is the fact that the pollen grain is quite strong. Each pollen grain has a double-walled husk of two parts, called the exine and intine, which surrounds the pollen food (cytoplasm). The outer wall, called the exine (sporopollen), is able to withstand strong acids and temperatures up to 300 degrees centigrade. Strengthening the pollen grain even further are various external resin deposits.

This makes the husk indigestible by the human body (unless treated or micronized), and further makes it possible for a pollen grain to last for thousands of years. Occasionally, a story will appear about seeds or pollen granules being found at an archaeological dig that are still biologically active. Some seeds found in the Egyptian pyramids have been planted and still germinated and grew after all these centuries.

G. Franchi and his team at the Institute of General Pathology, reported in 1996 that, of the pollens tested, it took a minimum of twelve hours for any of the pollen to be digested. Even at that, after 24 hours, some pollens showed only a 0.8-5.6% digestion rate. On average, after 24 hours only about 3% of the pollen food can be digested by humans from an intact pollen grain due to this strong double husk, and most of that is digested out through the pollen tube opening called the hila. This outer covering must be dissolved or broken to allow full digestibility of the pure cytoplasm inside. With the normal human digestion time of 12 hours, it is likely that almost none of the non-micronized pollen is digested and thus useable by the human body.[4]

It appears likely that 97% or more of unprocessed bee pollen remains undigested and unusable by the body.

It is simply swallowed and then excreted with little benefit in between.

It should be re-emphasized that the major problem with bee pollen is

---

> **"Swiss Micronized Flower Pollen... [is] the most concentrated nutrient-rich whole food in the world."**

---

not in the pollen itself, but rather the problems sometimes associated with the collection and storage methods used by the bee, not to mention pollen's almost total indigestibility. These conditions are of no consequence to the bee, but may be to humans. For people concerned about health and nutrition, the best possible pollen is certainly the most desirable.

SWISS MICRONIZED FLOWER POLLEN - THE "SUPER" POLLEN

Swiss micronized flower pollen is very different from ordinary bee pollen. First, a very unique proprietary natural process called micronization opens the pollen grain and exposes the pure pollen food, making it fully digestible by humans.

Then, Swiss pollen is pre-digested with live enzymes to make it hypoallergenic. These enzymes reduce the molecular size of the pollen, which removes harmful allergens. Allergic reactions are caused mainly by substances having a large molecular size. Enzyme predigestion reduces the molecular size of the pollen cytoplasm, making an allergic reaction highly unlikely.

Of great importance is the fact that the Swiss use absolutely no chemicals or solvents for this process. Some

TWO TYPES OF POLLEN

Cutaway of Unmicronized Pollen (husk intact)

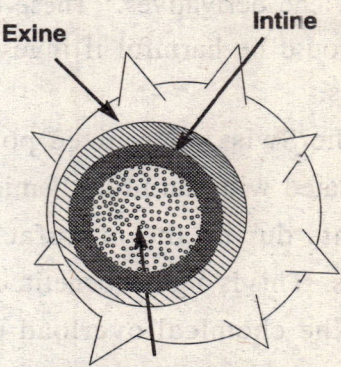

Unmicronized pollen is covered with an undigestible husk that prevents significant utilization of the valuable nutritionally-rich cytoplasm inside.

Relative Size and Consistency of Micronized Pollen

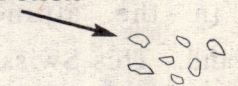

Micronizing the pollen makes the nutritional treasure inside more completely bioavailable.

other pollen processors treat the pollen with deadly chemicals, such as acetone or ethylene derivatives. These chemicals would be harmful if ingested by humans.

The Swiss micronized pollen is not treated with harmful chemicals or solvents during the manufacturing process. This is a great benefit, considering the chemical overload placed upon most humans today by a highly industrialized society and processed foods.

This micronized pollen is derived from a blend of eighty different pollens from flowers, grasses, and conifers grown in the alpine area of Switzerland. This Swiss pollen contains a broad spectrum of micronutrients that are very beneficial for humans.

TWO TYPES OF POLLEN

Swiss micronized pollen is thus a superior food supplement with a naturally balanced supply of important nutrients in concentrated form. It supplies these nutrients, which include essential amino acids, unsaturated fatty acids, enzymes, and various complex carbohydrates, vitamins, minerals, and trace elements directly to the body and cells. It also helps improve absorption of vital nutrients from the foods we eat, and facilitates better energy.

Made in Switzerland, the pollen is purified, processed and mixed with enzymes to break down the outer covering and reduce molecular weight of the pollen grains. Only pollen manufactured in this way can have such a greater value.

Swiss micronized pollen is pure food, and is easily digested by the body. Many believe it to be a concentrated nutrient-rich whole food. Pollen processed in this manner becomes a higher-grade pollen, containing vitamins, minerals, enzymes, protein, micronutrients, RNA, DNA, antioxidants, amino acids, flavonoids, carotinoids, natural hormones and other nutrients.

Nutritionally classified as a "Superfood," some nutritionists believe pollen to be a very important food. Swiss micronized pollen is far superior to normal bee pollen or even beehive royal jelly. The Swiss are very particular about cleanliness and their nutrient supplements, especially so in the formulation facility that processes Swiss pollen. Swiss micronized flower pollen is undoubtedly the highest-quality chemical-free pollen in the world.

Chapter 3
Pollen and the Prostate

By 40 years of age, 20-40% of men worldwide experience a benign enlargement of the prostate gland. By age 50, 68% of men in America suffer with this problem. By age 70, 80% of the men in industrialized nations are afflicted, while 99% of the men in China 70 years and older battle this problem.

The World Health Organization reports that 80% of men suffer from prostate problems at some point, and 33% of these will require surgery. For those men who contract prostate cancer, 37% will die from the disease.

The enlarged prostate exhibits various tell-tale characteristics, most notably that of restricting urine flow and poor emptying of the bladder. This occurs as the prostate gland increases in size and compresses the urinary tract. Other more irritating symptoms usually occur as well, such as pain while urinating, frequent daytime and sleep-robbing nighttime trips to the bathroom, urine hesitancy or poor urine flow, and loss of bladder control.

The most widely used medical treatment today is a surgical process called prostatectomy. Over 350,000 of these procedures are done every year in America. This surgery requires a hospital stay of several days, and a substantial recovery time.

Since the prostate is a secondary sex gland, hormonal drugs have been used to shrink and reduce inflammation. Hormonal inhibitors and neurological blockers are commonly prescribed. These drugs may often have unpleasant and undesirable side effects, especially in elderly patients.

Interestingly, prostate trouble is unknown in castrated males. Until the

> *"Pollen is used nutritionally throughout Europe and Asia to help solve prostatitis and prostate difficulties"*

late 19th century, castration was a recommended treatment for prostate enlargement. For obvious reasons, that treatment proved to not be very popular.

In Europe, many herbs and plants, under license to pharmaceutical-quality manufacturers, have been used to provide nutritional factors associated with solving problems of prostate enlargement. Swiss micronized pollen has been used for this purpose for over twenty-eight years.

Pollen has been considered an effective nutritional aid to help the prostate gland as reported in scientific studies. Additionally, there were no significant side effects. Pollen contains lycopene, beta-sitosterol and numerous flavonoids which have been studied to help the prostate.

Current research seems to indicate that the hormone 5-alpha-dihydrotestosterone is involved in prostate problems. Too much dihydrotestosterone may lead to the problems associated with benign prostatic hyperplasia. Pollen apparently affects the dihydrotestosterone pathway, and either limits production or helps flush it from the system, but more research is needed in this area.

POLLEN AND THE PROSTATE

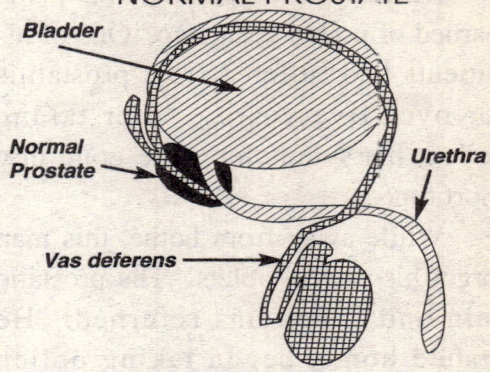

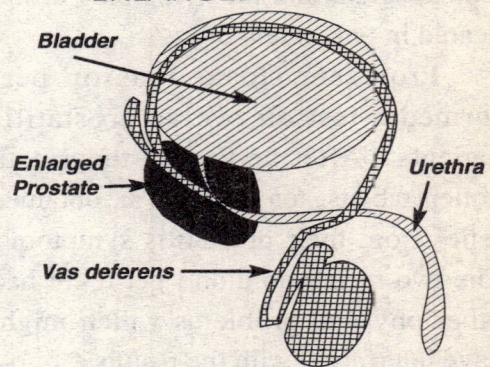

Over half of American men develop an enlarged prostate (Benign Prostatic Hyperplasia) as they approach their fifties. This swollen gland compresses the urethra and can cause a host of urinary and reproductive problems.

Dr. Erik Ask-Upmark, M.D., first learned of pollen years ago. One of his patients had suffered from prostatitis for over five years. After taking pollen, his symptoms were gone in a short time.

While away from home, this man forgot his pollen tablets. The prostatic pain and symptoms returned. He rushed home, began taking pollen tablets again, and the symptoms disappeared in only a few days.[2]

Professor Gosta Jonsson performed a test on twelve prostatitis patients. After he treated them with pollen tablets, ten men, 83%, obtained relief from their prostatitis symptoms. The two men who didn't get relief had other physical problems which might have interferred with the results.[2]

Dr. Ask-Upmark and Dr. Jonsson were among the very first researchers to establish a link between prostate relief and flower pollen.

Recent pharmacological studies and controlled clinical trials performed at prestigious university centers in England, Germany, Japan, Switzerland and Sweden show that flower pollen can have a significant nutritional effect on prostate enlargement and inflammation. These studies would indicate that pollen is as effective as most forms of pharmacological medication. Taken daily, pollen can help provide welcome nutritional symptomatic relief from frequent urinations and aid to reduce the amount of urine retained in the bladder.

Dr. A.C. Buck of the Department of Urology at the University Hospital of Wales, and his team of eight researchers, performed two very significant studies of pollen and the prostate gland.[5,6]

They noted that while surgical prostatectomy still remains a standard medical treatment for prostate obstruction, pharmacological intervention now appears to be an attractive alternative.

Notwithstanding the common desirability for medical treatment, most drugs used to treat prostate problems block the hormonal or neurological pathways, and it seems that all of the prostate drugs have undesirable side effects.

Feeling that flower pollen would possibly be of value, Dr. Buck and his associates performed a test to ascertain its benefit. The scientists developed a double-blind, placebo-controlled study to evaluate the effect of a six-month course of supplementation using flower pollen.

Test subjects were men who were on the waiting list for surgical prostate treatment. The results indicated a 69% success rate in those men using pollen. A subsequent study indicated a success rate for pollen of 78%.[7] Men with benign prostatic hyperplasia or mild to moderate outflow obstruction improved significantly.

It is important to note that while prostate hyperplasia takes several years to develop, the above test subjects

> **"69% [of men] with benign prostatic hyperplasia... or outflow obstruction improved significantly."**

experienced these success results in six months or less, and while taking only 240 mg of pollen per day. Dr. Buck surmised that a longer duration of treatment or a larger amount of pollen may produce a more pronounced benefit.

Additionally, following several reports that flower pollen was an effective agent for prostate problems, Dr. Buck undertook the following test.

This study showed that of the nine cell lines tested, the cell lines derived from human prostate were growth-inhibited by flower pollen, whereas the non-prostate cells showed varying degrees of resistance to the pollen. The positive effect of the pollen on prostate cell lines was even more pronounced in the hormone-independent models, suggesting that flower pollen might have a place in the control of abnormal growth in hormone-insensitive cells.

Simply stated, this study shows that flower pollen can nutritionally help with certain difficult prostate problems.

In Europe, pollen formulas have been used for years. Pharmacies and grocery stores routinely stock pollen as an over-the-counter nutrient supplement, especially for prostate problems. Pollen has been used nutritionally throughout Europe and Asia for years to help solve prostatitis and prostate difficulties.

Chapter 4

Pollen and Allergies

Pollen has been proven to help prevent or eliminate various symptoms of certain allergies. It has been tested for these benefits in Italy, Switzerland, China, Japan and Argentina, and has shown remarkable nutritional results under controlled clinical conditions.

Dr. Xiao Leng, M.D. of the Department of Allergy of the Peking Union Medical College Hospital, and a member of the Chinese Academy of Medical Sciences, led a team of three other doctors studying the effect of oral pollen immunotherapy on allergy patients.[8]

The test subjects received oral pollen supplementation for only twelve weeks. No systemic side effects were reported by any of the participants. All of the people receiving oral pollen supplements experienced a significant decrease in their allergic responses. They also reported relief from symptoms for up to three months after stopping the oral pollen treatments.

Of particular interest is the fact that none of the people receiving the placebo (fake) treatment in this double-blind study showed any improvement whatsoever in their allergic condition.

Dr. Leng reports that a similar study done by Dr. T.B. Tomasi demonstrated that it is possible to induce tolerance to many allergic substances simply by following a program of oral administration of pollen.[9] Dr. Leng reviewed over forty-one separate medical studies on pollen as well as performing the above study with his team of professional researchers.

Oral and sublingual immunotherapy has been used in Europe and also in the United States for many years, as reported by L.D. Dickey in the Journal of the American Medical Association.[10] More than 10 medical clinical trials have proven the beneficial effect of oral immunotherapy.[8] Oral administration of ragweed extracts has been used in the U.S. since the early 1900s to desensitize hayfever patients.[1]

The above reported scientific studies are a small portion of at least fifty-one studies on pollen and allergies which have reported favorable results in using pollen to help combat allergic reactions.

Certain allergies may be caused by fungi and bacteria on the outside of the pollen grain, and not the pollen itself. Swiss micronized pollen is hypoallergenic since it undergoes unique natural processes. It's an established doctrine of science that small and low molecular weight molecules, like Swiss micronized pollen, are generally not allergens. Swiss pollen also apparently works on helping relieve certain allergy symptoms by aiding the immune system in correcting whatever imbalance caused elevated histamine production in the first place. Through a phenomena known as persorption, some of the pollen ingested orally is believed to pass directly from the stomach into the bloodstream. This speeds up the process greatly, and accounts for the fact that pollen can be found in the blood, urine and spinal fluid within a few hours after ingestion.[3] Pollen-allergenic people should still consult their physician before beginning a pollen supplementation program, however.

Since it is free of harmful allergens and pesticide chemicals, even those who might be allergic to molds and bacteria occasionally found on bee pollen can better enjoy the benefits of Swiss pollen. For example, people highly allergic to hayfever allergens have taken Swiss micronized pollen without problems. It has actually helped reduce their hayfever symptoms.

Chapter 5

Pollen and Athletics

Pollen's greatest reputation is probably in the field of athletic and physical performance. Pollen's unique formula energizes the body to its maximum potential. Many world class athletes from various countries have increased their endurance and strength with pollen.

Dedicated weight lifters, runners, and body builders are discovering that pollen is a natural and safe substitute for very dangerous steroid drugs, with none of the side effects. Pollen is completely natural, and works with the body's physiology, not against it.

Pollen is widely used by European athletes, including the Finnish, Swedish, Russian and English national Olympic teams. They report that it increases training capacity, strength and stamina, accelerates transportation of nutrients to the cells, helps fight fatigue,

A famous Olympic coach reportedly gave pollen to his world-class gymnasts and expanded their anaerobic ability.

At the 1968 Olympic Games in Mexico, Finnish runners, who normally excel at long distance-running, failed to win any medals, and only one of their runners placed anywhere in the top 100. As a result, their trainers began a specialized program of supplementing their training diet with pollen.

POLLEN AND ATHLETICS

Finnish athletes began taking pollen. Athletes need good amounts of protein and a complete spectrum of

---

"Energy increased by 340% after only ten days, and went up hundreds of percent after ninety days."

---

amino acids for muscle repair. They found that they had more energy and were stronger while taking pollen. They could train longer and harder. The average daily run increased from 30 kilometres to 50 kilometres, an increase of 67%.[3]

After several years of using pollen, Lasse Viren, the Finnish long distance runner, ran in the 10,000 meter race in the 1972 Olympic Games. During the race, he lost his balance and fell to the ground. He got up and, despite the large lead of the other run-

---

"Endurance tests [with flower pollen] showed an increase of 263%."

---

ners, he had such immense reserve power that he overtook them and won the Gold Medal.[3] Even more amazingly, Viren repeated his win in the 1976 Olympic Games.[2]

In 1972, a conference was held in Sweden detailing the positive effects of flower pollen. Nine doctors from the Italian football teams reported on the use of pollen by nine of their teams.[3]

They stated that energy increased by 340% in only ten days, and ultimately increased exponentially by hundreds of percent. Oxygen capacity increased more than threefold, and endurance increased 163%. Thus energy, oxygen capacity and endurance all showed very significant increases.[12]

Reportedly, a famous Olympic coach gave pollen to his world-class and Gold medal gymnasts. It is known that pollen has been used by such persons as Muhammad Ali, Finnish Olympic distance running champion Lasse Viren, and comedian-turned-health activist, Dick Gregory. As a result of their good success with pollen in the 1972 Olympic Games, Finland gave pollen supplements to more than 1,000 of their Olympic athletes for the 1976 Olympic Games.[2]

Pollen is an energy supplement used by professional athletes to increase capacity, strength and stamina in training and competition. It acts to accelerate the transportation of nutrients to the cells, helps boost vitality, speeds energy recovery time, fights fatigue, and expands anaerobic ability. It also works as an ideal energy pick-me-up.

One study conducted in Scandinavia on flower pollen by M. Krotkiewski and a team of pollenologists found that muscle pain and soreness was noticeably reduced post-exercise, as well as finding almost a 39% reduction in lactic acid production. Also, glycogen levels in the muscle were increased. All this points to a large improvement in the level of sports ability.[13]

Chapter 6
Pollen and Good Health

Clinics in dozens of countries have used flower pollen for a wide variety of conditions of ill health.

A key to optimal health is found within the metabolic processes of the body's cells — proper assimilation of nutrients and elimination of wastes. That is how the cell can regenerate itself, continually building new cells according to the genetic code of the RNA/DNA in the cell nucleus. Since pollen is an ideal food for vitalizing cell functions, activating metabolism, and "feeding" genetic RNA/DNA replication according to the cellular blueprint, it follows that it is an ideal food for optimal nutritional health.

Pollen is truly a "glandular rocket fuel." The endocrine glands regulate various systems of the body by secreting small amounts of hormones. Virtually all the precursors to these hormones are found within flower pollen. By supplying a wide spectrum of micronutrients for cell metabolism and glandular function, pollen supports the self-regulatory functions of the body for optimal health.

A natural benefit of such optimal health is more energy. For many people, pollen can provide new vim, vigor, and vitality. Swiss micronized pollen allows the body to exhibit more of its vivacious feminine glow or powerful masculine virility.

Pollen has a good antioxidant effect. It helps deactivate or destroy free radicals created during the course

---

CHART 1
Summary of the Benefits of Pollen

- Helps stimulate body defense mechanisms.
- Can produce an anti-inflammatory effect.
- Seems to assist immuno-stimulation.
- Assists the body's physiological defenses.
- Can give added release of natural energy.
- Helps facilitate the ATP/ADP energy cycle.
- Antioxidant
- Assists in natural cellular regeneration.
- Helps body release untapped energy from ATP cycle
- Based on 30 years of experience using revolutionary technology

of normal cellular activity, or those caused by smoking or eating dark-roasted foods, such as coffee. Antioxidant activity helps protect cells in vital organs against harmful effects caused by toxic substances in the environment and food.

In addition, pollen appears to contain a group of nutritional components which are useful in helping the liver detoxify itself from harmful and toxic substances.

The main benefits of Swiss micronized flower pollen are these: it carries nutrients to the cells, boosts energy, supplies vitamins and minerals, acts as an antioxidant, helps the body adapt to stress, reduces platelet aggregation, helps stimulate the body's natural self-defense system, helps low serum lipid level, aids control of prostaglandin synthesis, and aids in liver detoxification.

It is possible that many of pollen's significant benefits are due to its levels

> *"Pollen has also been found to aid in both weight gain and weight loss."*

of bioflavonoids and phenolic acid derivatives. Bioflavonoids are powerful antioxidants, and have been linked to nutritionally helping many of the body's systems fight off various problems.

Another likely source of Swiss micronized pollen's exceptional nutritional value is that it contains both pollen and pollen fiber. Recently, pollen researchers have linked pollen fiber to increased fighting power in the immune system. While other pollen must have processed fiber added to it, Swiss pollen has always contained good amounts of pollen fiber from a widely-mixed variety of plants. Swiss pollen fiber undergoes the same natural micronization as the pure pollen cytoplasm for maximum bioavailability. Thus, this pollen formulation provides powerful benefits as it contains monocotyledon, dicotyledon and conifer pollen food, as well as monocotyledon, dicotyledon and conifer pollen fiber.

Two of the most interesting studies done recently on pollen were conducted by J. Zhao of the Shanghai Institute of Hemotology at the Shanghai Medical University in China. His team of nine researchers studied a

Traditional Chinese Medicine called pollen typhae, and reported their results in the prestigious American medical journal, Thrombosis Research.[14,15]

Pollen typhae remedy is a pollen taken from the Typha angustifolia L. plant. Their research found that this pollen has an antiatherosclerotic effect, and that its benefits are actually multiplied by various biological components found within the pollen itself. They concluded that pollen typhae has the effect of alleviating clinical symptoms of certain heart problems.

They also found that platelet aggregation was reduced significantly. The flavonoids in pollen typhae demonstrate an antiatherogenic action as well. This study, quoting a pollen study done by J. Wojcicki, noted that pollen could lower serum cholesterol level, inhibit platelet aggregation and promote vessel wall production of prostacyclin.[16]

> *"Pollen is truly a 'glandular rocket fuel'"... virtually all precursors to hormones are found within flower pollen."*

In general, pollen helps maintain bodily reactivity and flexibility and aids to help regulate the metabolic processes and levels for well-being.

Sir Alec Isaac, the Englishman who discovered Interferon, studied pollen for two years. Interferon is an anti-viral and disease-fighting substance in the body. Amino acids in pollen are readily absorbed by the body, and are used by the body to build

Interferon. Isaac found that pollen not only penetrates the wall of the cell, but also penetrates the cell membrane. It then combines with cell RNA and DNA and synthesizes interferon for use by the body's immune system. Much scientific interest has arisen concerning Interferon over the last few years.

POLLEN AND CHILD BEARING

Pollen, as the male cell of the plant kingdom, has a well-deserved reputation for extra vim, vigor, and virility. It provides all the biofactors that are precursors for the male and female hormones, and micro-nutrients essential for healthy reproductive systems. Reportedly, exclusive animal breeders in Europe pay top dollar for pollen concentrates that are added to their animals' food.

Some couples have reported increased libido and increased fertility. Today, flower pollen is a superfood source used by some doctors to help remedy certain dietary deficiencies associated with certain problems of the reproductive system.

Chapter 7
Scientific Information on Pollen

Pollen is perhaps the most unique creation of the natural world. It cannot be synthesized in a laboratory. Each pollen grain is distinct, in that it carries a fingerprint of it's own species. It contains all the substances needed for plant growth and thus is the basis for the entire food chain. Pollen guarantees the survival of the plant world, and is an essential part of the human life cycle. Plant life begins with fertilization by microscopic pollen grains. It takes about 6 grains to be seen by the human eye. Some of the largest pollens are so minute that it takes 400,000 grains to weigh one ounce. The smaller pollen grains require eight million grains to weigh one ounce.[3]

Plants grow, and animals eat them for food. It could be argued, and quite reasonably, that life on earth would cease without pollen. Plants would not germinate, and animals and man would have no food to sustain themselves. Without pollen, man and animals could die of starvation.

Detailed chemical composition of pollen was not known until the 1980s. It was found that pollen has more important biofactors than perhaps any other substance known to man. Scientists have identified all 22 amino acids, 27 mineral salts, all vitamins including A, C, D, and B complex and many enzymes and coenzymes in pollen. It contains more than 25 trace elements. Pollen is rich in carotenoids, bioflavonoids and phytosterols. Some researchers believe that it contains every substance needed to maintain life.

The highly complex pollen molecule is a rich wide-spectrum source of amino acids, short peptides, nucleic acids (RNA & DNA), vitamins, minerals, trace elements, fatty acids, phytosterols, terpenes, aliphatic alcohols, flavonoids, coenzymes, and prostaglandin precursors found in nature. In total, pollen contains well over 100 biologically-active nutritional components.

Pollen's various components act as catalysts, utilizing natural food values that could normally be lost.

Research done at the Institute of Medicine at the Zhejiang Academy of

Medical Sciences demonstrated that twenty percent pollen increases plaque and specific rosette-forming cells associated with an improved physiological response to invader cells, as well as reducing the liperoxide levels in brain, liver and blood serum.[17] Drs. Ockerman, Wojcicki and Samochowiec reported that pollen helped lower the levels of serum cholesterol and low density lipoproteins (LDL) while increasing the levels of "good" cholesterol (HDL).[18]

Due to its nutritional composition, pollen has also been associated with improved digestion and aiding longevity. It has been reported that a substantial percentage of older people in more remote parts of the world have been beekeepers. Typically, they kept the darkest (pollen-rich) honey at the bot-

SCIENTIFIC INFORMATION ON POLLEN

tom of the beehive for themselves. While this bee pollen was inferior to today's Swiss pollen, it nonetheless provided some nutritional benefits. Swiss micronized pollen is pure, non-allergenic and meets pharmaceutical-grade manufacturing standards. Due to these stringent controls, there is little variation from one bottle to the next.

As our other research details, cell mitochondria help create ATP from Q10, ADP, fats and carbohydrates. When the cell needs energy, it takes ATP and converts it to ADP, releasing energy in the process. Pollen helps the cells release a maximum amount of energy during the ATP cycle. In so doing, the cells and body are energized.

Once offered to Americans in only a chemically extracted form, pollen is now available in a pure and natural product. This newer formulation represents an important scientific advance in pollen research for a more pure, potent, and perfected flower pollen.

Until 1970, natural micronized flower pollen did not exist. In 1970, natural micronized pollen was developed using enzymatic pre-digestion for an astoundingly different and superior pollen product. These pollen products have seen widespread use and success in Europe.

Scientific testing in the U.S. in the 1980s found that pollen is a potent antioxidant.

Noting that pollen has been used as a food source for thousands of years, this testing demonstrated that pollen matches vitamin E in its antioxidant power.

This is a significant finding given the large amount of scientific data regarding the efficacy of vitamin E and its ability to correct nutritional deficiencies associated with some rather serious conditions of ill health.

Of further interest is that this testing also demonstrated that pollen extracts are proper and efficacious for supplemental nutritional use.

Chapter 8
The History of Flower Pollen

The researcher who discovered pollen's many benefits was a beekeeper. He developed a process to harvest pollen to feed to his bees. He found that by feeding pollen to the bees, the queen would lay more eggs, and the hive would produce more honey.

Even in these very beginning days of pollen research, it was noted that pollen caused the queen bee to be more fertile. Years later, human users of flower pollen would anecdotally report that pollen seemed to increase human fertility and allow them to have more children.

As pollen research continued, scientists discovered that bees use pollen to make royal jelly. The royal jelly is fed to only a few bee larvae, who later become the queens of the colonies. With three times the size, and ten times the life span of the other bees, the queen owes it all to one thing — a diet of highly synthesized pollen.

But research didn't stop there. Man went on to discover how to remove the pure pollen food (cytoplasm) from the hard double-walled resinous husk (exine and intine) surrounding it. Bees, when making royal jelly, use substances from their mandibular and hypopharyngeal glands to extract the pollen food from inside the grain.

Taking their cues from the bees, Swiss pollen researchers developed a natural and chemical-free process to break open the membrane of the pollen grain, making the pure pollen food available for human digestion.

Pollen contains molecules of both high- and low-molecular weight. Since the higher molecular weight substances may cause allergic reactions in some individuals, a natural enzyme process was developed to break apart these substances and make them more bioavailable. The result is a pollen that is more readily absorbed into the body.

Dr. Leander M.D., a urologist, tested 179 patients with prostate problems using a double-blind protocol. He found that pollen increased the recovery rate of his patients when compared to traditional treatments by as much as 80%, and sometimes as high as 92%.[2]

Tests in France showed that pollen was effective for use by eating disorder sufferers. It was very nourishing and allowed them to normalize their weight.

CHART 2
Comments from Pollen Users

One or more of the following:

- More positive mental outlook
- Increased feeling of well-being
- Less sleep required
- Higher energy levels
- Increased ability to accomplish work
- More alert
- Better athletic performance
- Improved digestion and nutrient assimilation

Pollen was registered in France for this use.[3]

Pollen is used as a nutritional remedy for prostate problems throughout Europe, Asia, Africa, Scandinavia, England and the Middle East. Researchers have found that pollen has a beneficial effect on cell metabolism.

In many countries throughout the world, flower pollen is prescribed by doctors or pharmacists for various health reasons.

Over the last twenty-eight years, Swiss researchers have led a team of pollenologists to unlock the secrets of life stored in this potent superfood. Used by numerous Olympic champions and health-conscious families in many countries of the world for years, Swiss micronized flower pollen should be a staple in everyone's dietary plan or program.

Chapter 9
Clinical Studies and Anecdotal Reports

IMPORTANT NOTE: In addition to the authoritative studies presented elsewhere in this book, the following anecdotal reports are presented for your review. Anecdotal reports are not valid for making scientific or categorical statements about the efficacy of any substance.

ALLERGIES

Dr. Urs Lenggenhager performed a test on his patients using Swiss micronized pollen. It was very successful, and the pollen caused no allergic reaction.

PROSTATE COMPLAINTS

The effect of pollen on the enlarged prostate has been tested in two urological clinics in Upsala and Lund, Sweden. Very positive results were achieved with the daily consumption of pollen. The Spanish physician Dr. Guemez Diaz has reported success using pollen in cases of prostate vesiculitis. The Romanian urologist, Dr. Roman, gave pollen to 34 patients, ranging in age from 56 to 75, with enlarged prostate. In addition to pollen, other beekeeping products were prescribed (propolis and royal jelly). On completion of the testing, the patients reported that they felt better and experienced a decreased urge to urinate, and the physician diagnosed diminished prostate enlargement.[19]

ARTERIOSCLEROSIS, CHOLESTEROL

According to the Romanian physician Dr. Georgescu, the consumption of pollen by his patients led to a decrease in their cholesterol and beta lipoprotein levels.[19]

ACNE AND SKIN PROBLEMS

Dr. Lars-Erik Essen of Sweden reports that a pollen preparation he formulates helps many people with acne and wrinkle problems, as well as promotes healthy and younger looking skin. Quoting Dr. Essen, "It seems to prevent premature aging of the cells and stimulates the growth of new skin tissue. It offers effective protection against dehydration and injects new life into dry cells. It smooths away wrinkles and stimulates the life-giving blood supply to all cells."[2]

MUSCLE INCREASE, CARDIOVASCULAR SYSTEM

A group of athletes in Romania received a daily amount of pollen and honey in addition to their standard

3500 calorie diet. The general condition of these athletes showed improvement only 4 days after treatment, and their enthusiasm for training increased. Within 10 days, their body weight increased between 0.4 and 1.7 kg, without an increase in fat tissue. A positive influence on heart function and recovery pulse, as well as improved oxygen uptake, was measured. Both the curve showing increasing strength and metabolic tests showed a more efficient use of energy. The physicians spoke in this connection of the general, bio-stimulating effect of pollen and honey.[19]

INFECTIONS

In a Swedish clinical experiment, Professor Olav Lindahl reported the protective effect of pollen against infections of the upper respiratory system.[20]

STRENGTHENING EFFECT

Extensive documentation has been gathered in France on the strengthening effect of pollen in patients with a variety of diseases.[20]

BONE FRACTURES

More rapid healing takes place in bone fractures in animals when they are given pollen.[20]

GERIATRICS

Humans over 70 years of age given pollen show weight increase, improved appetite, reduced fatigue and improvement in various blood values.[20]

Dr. Franziska Stengel gave Swiss micronized pollen to older patients, noting the following results:

- Increased physical activity
- Increased energy
- More restful sleep
- More rapid hair growth

- Increased work load
- Improved intestinal health

No conflict with any medication was noted.

COLDS AND INFLUENZA

The Swedish physician Dr. Stephen Mark-Vendel has reported on more than 300 families which suffered from chronic colds from fall until spring. Treated with pollen, 75-80% of these adults and children showed no illnesses in winter, year after year.[20]

Dr. Klapsche of Sweden conducted a trial using pollen against a flu epidemic. Of the 510 people tested, 98% remained free from flu symptoms.

PEDIATRICS

Dr. Stephen Mark-Vendel, senior consultant at the state pediatric clinic in southern Sweden, reports on his extensive practical clinical experience with

THE HISTORY OF POLLEN EXTRACT

pollen. In 1957 he received 95 calls in a 6 week period regarding children ill with severe cases of Hong Kong flu.

Hospitalization of these children would normally have been necessary. At first he treated them with the usual medications and vitamin C, without marked improvement. Then he gave the children flower pollen in addition, whereupon improvement without fever was noted in less than 48 hours. In similar cases, treated without pollen, his colleagues in the same city did not achieve the same results. In cases of measles and chicken pox, the disease lasted only 24-36 hours, and no complications were noted.

Dr. Mark-Vendel has used pollen therapy in his practice in Sweden in 600 cases, and has never noted any side effects.[20]

ANAEMIA

Professor Remy Chauvin from France noted in the year 1946 that anaemic children improved when given pollen, and that the iron in their blood increased.[21]

The same successful results have been reported by Russian researchers in humans, and by Romanian researchers in mice.[19]

CONSTIPATION

Professor Remy Chauvin also discovered the intestinal regulating effect of pollen.[21]

LIVER DISEASE (HEPATITIS)

A team of Romanian doctors gave 110 patients with chronic hepatitis pollen every day for 90-180 days. Laboratory tests showed an improvement in the ratio of blood albumin to gamma globulin in every patient. In a concurrent animal experiment, 60 laboratory mice were treated with carbon tetrachloride, which causes hepatitis. Feeding these ill animals pollen caused a marked improvement in measurable blood protein values.[19]

RADIATION THERAPY

At the University Women's Clinic in Vienna, Austria, Professors Weghaupt and Gitsch, together with a team of physicians, carried out an experiment with pollen in 25 patients receiving radiation therapy. Fifteen patients received a pollen diet, ten women received no pollen. The professors reported that extensive blood enzyme tests showed a visible decrease in the side effects of radiation in those patients receiving pollen. Their comment, "We see the marked effectiveness of a pollen diet shown both subjectively and in laboratory findings."[22]

CLINICAL TESTING

Dr. Zelimir Pavkovic of the People's Health Centre in Zagreb has used Swiss micronized pollen on many patients, noting the following results:

- Increased energy
- Increased strength
- Finger tremors ceased
- Depression eliminated
- Menstrual pain eliminated
- Headaches reduced or eliminated
- Bronchial problems helped
- Better sleep
- Increased calmness
- Cramps eliminated
- Libido increased
- Appetite improved
- Forgetfulness decreased

- Better circulation in extremities
- Better digestion
- Reduced constipation

MEDICAL SYMPOSIUM

At the Medical-Pharmaceutical Congress of 1978 in Florence, Professor Olav Lindahl of the medical faculty in Linkoping, Sweden, reported the following positive characteristics of pollen:

- Pollen does not damage the fetus in utero.
- Pollen is not toxic.
- Animals given pollen heal more quickly and show an improved immune system.
- In laboratory tests, red blood cells are destroyed by the bactericide, strepolysin. In blood mixed with pollen

extract, the red blood cells are
not destroyed by the
bactericide.

APPENDIX A

A Chemical Analysis of Nutritional Factors in Flower Pollen

(as contained naturally and in varying amounts)

—— VITAMINS ——

- Provitamin A (Carotenoids)
- B Vitamins
- B1 Thiamine
- B2 Riboflavin
- B3 Niacin
- B6 Pyridoxine
- Rutin
- Biotin
- B12
- Vitamin C
- Vitamin D
- Vitamin E
- Vitamin K
- Choline
- Folic Acid
- Inositol
- Pantothenic Acid

—— MINERALS ——

- Boron
- Calcium
- Chromium
- Copper
- Iodine
- Iron
- Magnesium
- Manganese
- Molybdenum
- Phosphorus
- Potassium
- Silicon
- Sodium
- Sulphur
- Titanium
- Zinc

—— CAROTENOIDS ——

- Beta-carotene
- Crocetin
- Lycopene
- Xanthophylls
- Zeaxanthin

AMINO ACIDS
(DIETARY ESSENTIAL)

- Histidine
- Isoleucine
- Leucine
- Lysine
- Methionine
- Phenylalanine
- Threonine
- Tryptophan
- Valine

AMINO ACIDS
(PHYSIOLOGICALLY ESSENTIAL)

- Alanine
- Alpha-Amino-Butyric-Acid
- Arginine
- Asparagine
- Aspartic Acid
- Cystine
- Glutamic Acid
- Glutamine
- Glycine
- Hydroxyproline
- Proline
- Serine
- Tyrosine

PROSTAGLANDINS

A group of hormone-like compounds derived from linoleic and arachidonic acids that influence innumerable body processes.

PHYSTOSTEROLS

- Fucosterol
- Campesterol
- Beta-sitosterol
- Estrone
- Stigmasterol

APPENDIX A

—— ENZYMES ——

24 Oxidoreductases
21 Transferases
32 Hydrolases
10 lyases

5 Isomerases
2 Ligases and
Others

—— FATTY ACID PROFILE ——
(Number of C-atoms and double bonds)

Caprylic (C-6)
Capric (C-10)
Lauric (C-12)
Myristic (C-14)
Myristoleic (C-14) 1 dbl. bond
Pentadecanoic (C-15)
Pentadecenoic (C-15) 1 dbl. bond
Palmitic (C-16)
Palmitoleic (C-) 1 dbl. bond
Heptadecanoic (C-17)
Heptadecenoic (C-17) 1 dbl. bond
Stearic (C-IX)
Oleic (C-13) 1 dbl. bond
Linoleic (C-13) 1 dbl. bond
Linolenic (C-13) 2 dbl. bonds
Arachidic (C-20)
Eicosenoic (C-20) 1 dbl. bond
Eicosadienoic (C-20) 2 dbl. bonds
Eicosadienoic (C-20) 3 dbl. bonds
Arachidonic (C-20) 4 dbl. bonds

LOW MOLECULAR WEIGHT SUGARS
— AND RELATED COMPOUNDS —

- Fructose
- Glucose
- Mannose
- Xylose
- Galactose
- Xylitol
- Arabinose
- Xylogalacturonan
- Ribose
- Glucoronolactone
- Fucose
- Raffinose
- Hexasamine
- Stachyose
- Rhamnose
- Sucrose
- Maltotetratose
- Maltose
- Maltotriose
- Callose

—— FLAVONOIDS ——

- Quercetin
- Apigenin
- Kaempferol
- Dihydroxquercertin
- Narigenin
- Myricetin
- Luteolin
- Isorhamnetin

LONG CHAIN
—— HYDROCARBONS ——

- n-pentacosane
- Myo-inositol
- n-heptacosane
- Pinitol
- n-nonacosane
- Sequitol
- n-tricosane

—— GROWTH REGULATORS ——

- Auxins
- Brassins
- Gibberellins
- Kinins

APPENDIX A

DIFFERENT CLASSES OF LIPIDS
—— IN FLOWER POLLEN ——

The major fractions of the polar lipids in flower pollen are lecithin, lysolecithin, phosphoinositol and phosphatidylcholine.

NATURAL LIPIDS

- Monoglycerides
- Diglycerides
- Triglycerides
- Free fatty acids
- Sterols
- Hydrocarbons

OTHERS

- Chlorophyll
- Guanine
- Nucleic Acids
- Amines
- Phenolic Acids
- Hexodecanal
- Vanillie
- Gallic
- P. coumaric
- Ferulic
- Protocatechuic
- Pentosans
- P. hydroxybenzoic Terpenes
- Nucleosides Vernine
- Xanthine
- Hypoxanthine
- Nuclein

UNKNOWN NUTRIENTS

Some of the nutritional values of Flower Pollen may stem from nutritional factors which are not fully researched by science, and from the synergistic action of all the factors working together. These factors may constitute additional life-enhancing powers of flower pollen.

APPENDIX B
Average nutritional value of pollen

Chemical	Composition	% of RDA/EDI
Energy	2.46 kcal/g[b]	
Protein	23.7%	420
Carbohydrates	27.0%	83
Lipids	4.8%	59[c]
Cholesterol	~0	~0[c]
Phosphorus	0.53%	590
Potassium	0.58%	190
Calcium	0.225%	250
Magnesium	0.148%	470
Sodium	0.044%	27[c]
Iron	140 ppm	830
Manganese	100 ppm	2500
Zinc	78 ppm	580
Copper	14 ppm	560
Nickel	4.5 ppm	[d]
Boron	trace	[d]
Chromium	?	?
Molybdenum	?	?
Iodine	?	?
Fluoride	?	?
Selenium	?	?
Thiamin	9.4 ppm	760
Niacin	157 ppm	940

Riboflavin	18.6 ppm	1300
Pyridoxine	9 ppm	500
Pantothenate	28 ppm	450
Folic acid	5.2 ppm	2600
Biotin	0.32 ppm	440
Vit. B_{12}	0	0
Vitamin C	350 ppm	520
Vitamin A	0	0 [e]
Carotenes	95 ppm	~900 [e]
Vitamin D	0	0
Vitamin E	14 ppm	160
Vitamin K	0	0

---

[a] Calculations based on RDA (Recommended Daily Allowance) and EDI (Estimated Daily Intake = Estimated Safe and Adequate Daily Dietary Intakes) using U.S. women aged 25-50 with a 2200 kcal intake (1).

[b] Calculated on the basis of 4 kcal/g for protein and carbohydrates, and 9 kcal/g for fat (28).

[c] These values are recommended maximum intakes for nutrients generally accepted as harmful to health in excess (1).

[d] Nutritional requirements in the human diet not established.

[e] Pollen contains no preformed Vit. A, but carotenes can be converted to Vit. A equivalents based on 6 µg ß-carotene = 1 Vit. A equivalent and assuming half pollen carotenes are ß-carotene.

APPENDIX B

Nutritional comparison of pollen and typical nutritious foods[a]

Food[b]	Protein (g)	Fat (g)	Potassium (g)	Calcium (mg)	Sodium (mg)	Iron (mg)
Pollen	96.3	19.5	2.4	915	179	57.0
Tomato	50.0	8.8	11.0	588	138	22.0
Cabbage	54.1	8.3	2.4	2037	835	16.0
Chicken	152.8	35.9	2.0	60	484	8.9
Beans	40.1	6.5	1.7	443	3800	15.0
Apple	3.4	10.3	1.9	122	19	5.3
Bread	43.2	12.3	1.1	407	2200	12.0
Beef	59.4	82.7	0.7	26	145	7.5

Continued on next page

92   SWISS MICRONIZED FLOWER POLLEN

Food[b]	Vit. A (Int. U)	Thiamin (mg)	Riboflavin (mg)	Niacin (mg)	Vit. C (mg)	Rank Score[c]
Pollen	14500	3.82	7.56	63.8	142	62
Tomato	41000	2.75	1.88	31.2	1050	60
Cabbage	5410	2.11	2.75	12.8	1950	58
Chicken	484	0.28	1.29	57.7	0	31
Beans	1070	0.65	0.25	4.9	16	30
Apple	1560	0.53	0.34	1.9	68	27
Bread	trace	1.06	0.49	11.5	trace	23
Beef	143	0.17	0.46	12.2	0	17

[a]All values are based on amount in the quantity of food that provides 1000 kcal of energy; data for the foods and for pollen calculated based on the values in Appendix C.
[b]Fresh raw tomato, cabbage, apple; fried chicken leg and breast; baked beans; whole wheat bread; broiled sirloin beef steak.
[c]Each food is ranked from 7 (highest nutrient content) to 0 (lowest nutrient content) for each of the 11 nutrient categories. Because increased dietary levels of fat and sodium are considered detrimental to health, the rankings are reversed (7=lowest; 0=highest) for these two nutrients. Rank score is the total of the 11 rankings for each food (lowest possible score=0; highest=77). The authors gratefully thank Dr. Justin O. Schmidt of the U.S. Department of Agriculture for providing the information contained in Appendix B, and Plenum Press, New York for allowing us to reprint this important data on pollen.

REFERENCES

1. Mizrahi, Avshalom and Lensky, Yaacov, "Bee Products: Properties, Applications and Apitherapy", Plenum Press, New York, 1997.
2. Wade, Carlson, "Bee Pollen and Your Health", Keats Publishing, Connecticut, 1978.
3. Hanssen, Maurice, "The Healing Power of Pollen", Thorsons Publishers, Wellingborough, England, 1979.
4. Franchi, G. G. et al., "Microspectrophotometric evaluation of digestibility of pollen grains", Plant Foods for Human Nutrition, 50: 115-126, 1997.
5. Buck, A., et al., "Treatment of outflow tract obstruction due to benign prostatic hyperplasia with the pollen extract, cernilton. A double-blind, placebo-controlled study", British Journal of Urology, 66(4):398-404, 1990.
6. Habib, F., et al., "In vitro evaluation of the pollen extract, cernitin T-60, in the regulation of prostate cell growth", British Journal of Urology, 66(4):393-7, 1990.
7. Rugendorff, E.W., W. Weidner, L Ebeling and A.C. Buck, "Results of Treatment with Pollen Extract (Cernilton N) in Chronic Prostatitis and Prostatodynia", British Journal of Urology 71, 433-438, 1993.
8. Leng, X., et al., "A double-blind trial of oral immunotherapy for Artemisis pollen asthma with evaluation of bronchial response to the pollen allergen and serum-specific IgE antibody", Annals of Allergy, 64(1):27-31, 1990.

9. Tomasi, T., "Oral tolerance", Transplantation, 29:353, 1980.
10. Dickey, L., "Sublingual antigens", Journal of the American Medical Association, 217:214, 1971.
11. Curtis, H., "The immunizing cure of hay fever", Medical News, p. 74., 1900.
12. Asplund, Ake, "Searching the Source of Life and Vitality", Sanomin (SA) SDN, Singapore, 1991.
13. Krotkiewski, M., et al., "Prevention of muscle soreness by pretreatment with antioxidants", Scand. Journal of Med. Sci. Sports 4:191-199, 1994.
14. Zhao, J., et al., "The antiatherogenic effects of components isolated from pollen typhae", Thrombosis Research, 57(6):957-66, 1990.
15. Zhao, J., et al., "Further study of pollen typhae's effects on the production of tPA and PGI, by cultured endothelial cells", Thrombosis Research, 56(6):677-85, 1989.
16. Wojcicki, J., et al., "Effect of pollen extract on the development of experimental atherosclerosis in rabbits", Atherosclerosis, 62:39-45, 1986.
17. Qian, B., et al., "Effects of bee pollen on lipid peroxides and immune response in aging and malnourished mice", China Journal Chinese Materia Medica, 15(5):301-3, 319, 1990.
18. Wojcicki, J., "Effect of pollen extract on the development of experimental atherosclerosis in rabbits, Atherosclerosis 62(1): 39-45, 1986.

19. Neues in der Apitherapie, II International Symposium, Apimondia Verlag, Bukarest, 1976.
20. Lindahl, Olav, "Proceedings of the Medical-Pharmaceutical Symposium -- 'Prevention is Better than the Cure'", Florence, 1978.
21. Chauvin, R., "Traite de Biologie de l'Abeille", Tome 3, Paris, 1968.
22. Hernus, P. et al., "Pollendiat als Adjuvans der Strahlentherapie", Strahlentherapie 150, 500-506, 1975.

BIBLIOGRAPHY/FURTHER READING

Ask-Upmark, E., *Prostatitis and its Treatment*, Acta Med. Scandinavia 181, 355-57, 1967.

Bell, R. R., E. J. Thornber, J. L. L. Seet, M. T. Groves, N. R. Ho and D. T. Bell, *Composition and Protein Quality of Honeybee-Collected Pollen of Eucalyptus calophylla*, Journal of Nutrition 113, 2479-2484, 1983.

Chauvin, R., *Traite de Biologie de l'Abeille, Tome 3*, Paris, 1968.

Denis, L. J., *Chronic Prostatitis*, Acta Urol. Belg. 34, 49-55, 1966. Hayashi, A. U., J. Mitsui, H. Yamakawa et al., Clinical Evaluation of Cernilton in Benign Prostatic Hypertrophy, Hinyokika Kiyo 32, 135-41, 1986.

Elkins, Rita, *Bee Pollen, Royal Jelly, Propolis and Honey*, Woodland Publishing, Pleasant Grove, 1996.

Hernus, P. et al., *Pollendiat als Adjuvans der Strahlentherapie*, Strahlentherapie 150, 500-

506, 1975.

Koch, A., and Schwarz, I., *Wirkstoffe der B-Gruppe in der Bienennahrung*, Congres' de l'Union Int. pour l'Etude des insectes Sociaux, Communications au IIe Congres Insectes Society, Wurzbourg 4, April 1955.

Murat, Dr. Felix,*Bee Pollen: Miracle Food*, Bee Wonderful, Edgewood, 1971.

Neues in der Apitherapie, II International Symposium, Apimondia Verlag, Bukarest, 1976.

Recommended Dietary Allowances, 10th Edition, National Academy Press, Washington. 1989.

Samochowiec, L., T. Dutkiewicz, J. Wojcicki and J. Gieldanowski, *The Influence of Pollen Extracts (Cernitin GBX and Cernitin T60) on Allergic Reactions*, Phytother. Res. 6, 314-317, 1992.

Schmidt, J.O. and S.L. Buchmann, *Other Products of the Hive, in: The Hive and the Honey Bee* (J.M. Graham, Editor), Dadant & Sons, Hamilton, IL 1992.

Schmidt, P. J., J. O. Schmidt and C. W. Weber, *Mesquite Pollen as a Dietary Protein Source for Mice*, Nutritional Reports International, 30, 513-22, 1984.

Wortmann, F., *Oral Immunotherapy*, Clin. Immunol. Allerg. 389-398, 1981.

Special note: The above Footnotes and Bibliography contain but a few of the many scientific references concerning pollen.